Petra Dickmann

Plague - Pandemic - Panic

Petra Dickmann

Plague - Pandemic - Panic

Information Needs and Communication Strategies for Infectious Diseases Emergencies

Südwestdeutscher Verlag für Hochschulschriften

Impressum/Imprint (nur für Deutschland/only for Germany)
Bibliografische Information der Deutschen Nationalbibliothek: Die Deutsche Nationalbibliothek verzeichnet diese Publikation in der Deutschen Nationalbibliografie; detaillierte bibliografische Daten sind im Internet über http://dnb.d-nb.de abrufbar.

Alle in diesem Buch genannten Marken und Produktnamen unterliegen warenzeichen-, marken- oder patentrechtlichem Schutz bzw. sind Warenzeichen oder eingetragene Warenzeichen der jeweiligen Inhaber. Die Wiedergabe von Marken, Produktnamen, Gebrauchsnamen, Handelsnamen, Warenbezeichnungen u.s.w. in diesem Werk berechtigt auch ohne besondere Kennzeichnung nicht zu der Annahme, dass solche Namen im Sinne der Warenzeichen- und Markenschutzgesetzgebung als frei zu betrachten wären und daher von jedermann benutzt werden dürften.

Verlag: Südwestdeutscher Verlag für Hochschulschriften GmbH & Co. KG
Dudweiler Landstr. 99, 66123 Saarbrücken, Deutschland
Telefon +49 681 37 20 271-1, Telefax +49 681 37 20 271-0
Email: info@svh-verlag.de

Approved by: Frankfurt, Universität, Diss. 2011

Herstellung in Deutschland:
Schaltungsdienst Lange o.H.G., Berlin
Books on Demand GmbH, Norderstedt
Reha GmbH, Saarbrücken
Amazon Distribution GmbH, Leipzig
ISBN: 978-3-8381-2629-6

Imprint (only for USA, GB)
Bibliographic information published by the Deutsche Nationalbibliothek: The Deutsche Nationalbibliothek lists this publication in the Deutsche Nationalbibliografie; detailed bibliographic data are available in the Internet at http://dnb.d-nb.de.

Any brand names and product names mentioned in this book are subject to trademark, brand or patent protection and are trademarks or registered trademarks of their respective holders. The use of brand names, product names, common names, trade names, product descriptions etc. even without a particular marking in this works is in no way to be construed to mean that such names may be regarded as unrestricted in respect of trademark and brand protection legislation and could thus be used by anyone.

Publisher: Südwestdeutscher Verlag für Hochschulschriften GmbH & Co. KG
Dudweiler Landstr. 99, 66123 Saarbrücken, Germany
Phone +49 681 37 20 271-1, Fax +49 681 37 20 271-0
Email: info@svh-verlag.de

Printed in the U.S.A.
Printed in the U.K. by (see last page)
ISBN: 978-3-8381-2629-6

Copyright © 2011 by the author and Südwestdeutscher Verlag für Hochschulschriften GmbH & Co. KG and licensors
All rights reserved. Saarbrücken 2011

PLAGUE – PANDEMIC – PANIC

INFORMATION NEEDS AND COMMUNICATION STRATEGIES FOR INFECTIOUS DISEASES EMERGENCIES
LESSONS LEARNED FROM ANTHRAX, SARS, PNEUMONIC PLAGUE AND INFLUENZA PANDEMIC

PETRA DICKMANN

FOR PAULA

CONTENTS

Summary	*Page 3*
Zusammenfassung	*Page 5*
Introductory Remarks	*Page 8*
Literature Review	*Page 11*
HOW TO REDUCE THE IMPACT OF 'LOW RISK PATIENTS' FOLLOWING A BIOTERRORIST INCIDENT: LESSONS LEARNED FROM SARS, ANTHRAX AND PNEUMONIC PLAGUE	
Appendix A: Search Strategy of the Literature Review	*Page 27*
Empirical Investigation	*Page 29*
NEW INFLUENZA A/H1N1 ("SWINE FLU"): INFORMATION NEEDS OF AIRPORT PASSENGERS AND STAFF	
Appendix B: Additional Material	*Page 44*
Passenger Questionnaire	*Page 44*
Staff Questionnaire	*Page 45*
Table 1-3: Demographics, Final Destinations, Fear Inbound/Outbound	*Page 46*
Figure 1: Information need: fear level and inbound/outbound flight	*Page 49*
Acknowledgements	*Page 51*

SUMMARY

Information and communication is critical to the successful management of infectious diseases because an effective communication strategy prevents the surge of anxious patients who have not been genuinely exposed to the pathogen ('low risk patients') affecting medical infrastructures (1) and the future transmission of the infectious agent (2).

Surge of low risk patients

The arrival of large numbers of low risk patients at hospitals following an infectious diseases emergency would be problematic for three main reasons. First, it would complicate the situation at hospitals receiving exposed patients, delaying the treatment of the acutely ill, creating difficulties of crowd control and tying up medical resources. Second, for the low risk patients themselves, attending hospital following an infectious disease emergency might increase their risk of exposure to the agent in question. Third, the needs of low risk patients may be poorly attended to at hospitals which are already overstretched dealing with medical casualties.

Future transmission

Obtaining early information about symptoms and isolating infected patients is the most effective strategy to interrupt the chain of infection in the public in the absence of specific prophylaxis or treatment. Particularly at the beginning of an outbreak, these non-pharmaceutical interventions play an important role in enabling the early detection of signs or symptoms and in encouraging passengers to adopt appropriate preventive behaviour in order to limit the spread of the disease.

This book includes two papers dealing with this problem:

The first part is a systemic literature review of information needs following an infectious disease emergency (Anthrax, SARS, Pneumonic Plague). The key question was: what are the information needs of the public during an infectious disease emergency?

The second part is an empirical investigation of information needs and communication strategies at the airport during the early stage of the Influenza Pandemic. The key question here was: what communication strategies help to meet the information needs and to enable the public to behave appropriately and responsibly?

Conclusions

Evidence from the anthrax attacks in the United States suggested that a surge of low risk patients is by no means inevitable. Data from the SARS outbreak illustrated that if hospitals are seen as sources of contagion, many patients with non-bioterrorism related health care needs may delay seeking help. Finally, the events surrounding the Pneumonic Plague outbreak of 1994 in Surat, India, highlighted the need for the public to be kept adequately informed about an incident to avoid creating rumours. Clear, consistent and credible information is key to the successful management of infectious disease outbreaks.

The results of the empirical investigation suggested that the desire for information is a reflection of current anxiety and does not mirror the objective scientific assessment of exposure. The airport study showed that perceived information needs were directly related to anxiety – the least anxious did not require any further information, the most anxious reported significant information needs concerning medical treatment, public health management and the assessment of the ongoing situation – irrespective of their actual exposure. A communication strategy only focussing on the 'real' exposed individuals neglects the information needs of those worrying about having contracted the virus and seeking medical attendance.

Effective communication strategies should enable the general public to detect early signs or symptoms and provide them with behaviour advice to prevent the further transmission of the infectious agent. These include the provision of clear information about the incident, the symptoms and what to do to prevent the further transmission, detailed and regularly updated information in various media formats (telephone, internet, etc.) and rapid triage at hospital entrances to guide patients to the appropriate medical infrastructures.

Relevance

These research findings could contribute to a shift in the organisational and communicative approach responding to infectious diseases outbreaks and could be considered relevant for future risk communication and policy decision-making.

Zusammenfassung

Information und Kommunikation sind die zentralen Momente im Management von Infektionskrankheiten, weil eine effektive Kommunikationsstrategie zum einen den Ansturm auf die medizinischen Infrastrukturen kanalisiert (1) und zum anderen durch die Informationen zum angemessenen Verhalten die weitere Übertragung des Krankheitserregers vermeidet (2).

Ansturm auf medizinische Infrastrukturen

Ein großer Ansturm von nicht direkt exponierten Patienten (sogenannte „Low Risk Patients") auf medizinische Infrastrukturen während Infektionsausbrüchen ist aus drei Gründen problematisch: Erstens verschärft dieser Ansturm die ohnehin schon schwierige Lage in den Krankenhäuser und führt dazu, dass Schwerkranke aus Kapazitätsgründen nicht angemessen versorgt werden können. Zweitens erhöht der Aufenthalt in der Notaufnahme eines Krankenhauses während eines Infektionsgeschehens die Infektionsgefährdung. Drittens ist durch die Kapazitätsausschöpfung nicht gewährleistet, dass „Low Risk Patients" entsprechend ihrer medizinischen Indikation adäquat versorgt werden.

Weitere Übertragung des Krankheitserregers

Die frühzeitige Information über Symptome, Übertragungswege und angemessenes Verhalten führt dazu, dass symptomatische Patienten isoliert und die weitere Verbreitung des Krankheitserregers durch ein adäquates Infektionsschutzverhalten gestoppt wird. Diese nicht-pharmazeutischen Maßnahmen sind insbesondere in der Frühphase von Infektionsausbrüchen, in denen noch keine Impfungen oder Therapien zur Verfügung stehen, von hoher Relevanz und helfen sowohl die symptomatischen Patienten zu identifizieren als auch die Bevölkerung mit einem angemessenen Verhalten zu schützen.

In diesem Buch werden zwei Arbeiten zusammengefasst, die dieser Problematik nachgehen: den ersten Teil bildet eine systematische Literaturübersicht über die publizierten Daten zu den Informationsbedürfnissen und zum adäquaten Verhalten während Infektionsausbrüchen am Beispiel von Anthrax, SARS und der Lungenpest. Leitfrage dieser Studie ist: Was sind die Informationsbedürfnisse der Öffentlichkeit während eines Infektionsgeschehens?

Den zweiten Teil bildet eine empirische Erhebung am Flughafen zu den Informationsbedürfnissen und Kommunikationsstrategien zu Beginn der Influenza Pandemie. Leitend bei dieser Studie ist die Frage, welche Kommunikationsstrategien den

Informationsbedürfnissen adäquat sind und gleichzeitig die Öffentlichkeit in die Lage versetzt, sich angemessen zu verhalten?

Ergebnisse

Die Anthrax Anschläge in den USA haben gezeigt, dass es nicht unbedingt zu einem Massenansturm von „Low Risk Patients" kommen muss, wenn die Informationen über Diagnostik und therapeutische Maßnahmen adäquat kommuniziert werden. Aus den Erfahrungen von SARS konnte man sehen, dass auch die umgekehrte Situation Probleme schafft: wenn Patienten, die medizinische Behandlung benötigen, nicht die medizinischen Infrastrukturen aufsuchen, weil diese selbst zum Ort der Ansteckung geworden sind, kann das dramatische medizinische Folgen haben. Der Ausbruch der Lungenpest in Indien, verknüpft in ein Netz von Gerüchten, hat deutlich gemacht, wie wichtig die umfassend und aktuell korrekt informierte Öffentlichkeit ist.

Die Ergebnisse aus der empirischen Arbeit am Flughaben belegen, dass das Informationsbedürfnis nicht an die wissenschaftlich-medizinische Einschätzung der Exposition und des objektiven Ansteckungsrisikos geknüpft ist, sondern vielmehr die *eigene Wahrnehmung* und das *Gefühl* einer möglichen Ansteckung reflektiert. Diejenigen, die am meisten Angst vor Ansteckung hatten, artikulierten auch den größten Informationsbedarf, während diejenigen, die sich ausreichend informiert fühlten, auch nur eine geringe Besorgnis zum Ausdruck brachten. Diese Relation wurde *unabhängig der objektiven Exposition* beobachtet. Eine Kommunikationsstrategie, die nur die objektiv Exponierten adressiert, zielt also an denjenigen vorbei, die – exponiert oder nicht – besorgt sind und aufgrund dieser Sorge zu einem Problem der medizinischen Infrastrukturen werden können.

Eine effektive Kommunikation sollte die Öffentlichkeit in die Lage versetzen, die entsprechenden Symptome frühzeitig zu erkennen und sich sowohl bei Erkrankung, als auch bei der Unterbrechung der Infektionskette adäquat zu verhalten. Dazu braucht es klare, aktuelle und glaubwürdige Informationen über das Ausbruchsgeschehen, die Symptome und das Schutzverhalten, kontinuierliche Kommunikation über verschiedene mediale Formate (Telefon, Internet, etc.), schnelle Triage in den Krankenhäusern und eine kompetente Führung, um festlegen zu können, welcher Patient in den spezifischen medizinischen Infrastrukturen am besten aufgehoben ist.

Relevanz

Die Ergebnisse dieser Arbeit können dazu betragen, dass eine verbesserte Risiko- und Krisenkommunikation das Management von Infektionskrankheiten der politischen Entscheidungsträger erleichtert.

INTRODUCTORY REMARKS

This book contains two articles (one published and one submitted) about the behaviour and information needs of the public in the context of an infectious disease emergency (IDE) caused by a deliberate release in a bioterrorist scenario (Anthrax), an emerging or re-emerging pathogen (SARS and Plague) or an Influenza pandemic. These incidents were chosen because they represent a matrix of incidents with enormous medical, social and economic impact: a bioterrorist attack, an emerging or re-emerging disease and a rapidly and globally spreading disease.

Systematic Literature Review

The first part of this book is a systematic literature review which assessed the impact of three outbreaks (Anthrax, SARS, Pneumonic Plague) on public behaviour in terms of attendance at healthcare facilities.

The key questions were: what is known about what the public wants to know? And: are there predictors of behaviour in response to infectious diseases outbreaks?

Method

A systematic search was made of Medline to identify publications that might contain data relevant to this review. A summary of the search strategy used is provided in Appendix A.

Papers were only selected for inclusion in this review if they:

- related to a general public sample (excluding, for example, studies of health care, emergency service or military personnel)
- related to one of the three outbreaks selected for study (Anthrax (2001 – "Amerithrax"), SARS (2003) or Pneumonic Plague in Surat/India (1994[1]) and
- contained relevant data concerning the prevalence of low risk patients, the predictors of health anxiety or behavioural response among low risk patients, or the information needs of low risk patients.

Papers were excluded if they consisted of:

- Exercises or hypothetical scenarios
- Articles published in languages other than English.

For the Anthrax and SARS outbreaks, papers expressing only expert opinion or anecdotal evidence were excluded. Given the paucity of relevant data that were available for the 1994

---

[1] The outbreak of Pneumonic Plague in Surat/India lasted from August 26, 1994 to October 18, 1994.

outbreak of pneumonic plague in Surat, however, for this incident such evidence was included where relevant.

The results of the review are presented narratively, broken down according to disease.

Organisational Remarks

This literature review was part of a programme of research being conducted by King's College London and the Health Protection Agency, entitled 'Behavioural Responses to Chemical, Biological, Radiological and Nuclear Incidents.' This research was funded under the Home Office CBRN Science and Technology Programme (study reference: 43/05/81). I was invited to take part in the research project while I was doing my medical elective period at the King's College Hospital, Institute of Psychiatry (Prof. Wessely), in March-April 2008. The research took place until September 2008 and we submitted the research report to the Home Office on October 1st, 2008. This literature review (Rubin & Dickmann: How to Reduce the Impact of 'Low Risk Patients' following a Bioterrorist Incident: Lessons Learned from SARS, Anthrax and Pneumonic Plague) was accepted for publication in December 2009 by the journal *Biosecurity and Bioterrorism. Biodefense Strategy, Practice, and Science* in their March issue.

Empirical Investigation

The second part of this book is an empirical investigation about the information needs of the public during an infectious disease emergency. With the beginning of the Influenza A/H1N1 epidemic (April 29-30, 2009) we conducted qualitative semi structured interviews at Frankfurt International Airport within the highest security zone of the primary security line of the gates[2] with passengers who were either returning from or going to Mexico and with airport staff who had close contact with these passengers. These interviews focused on knowledge about swine flu, information needs and anxiety concerning the outbreak. The aim of the study was to determine the adequacy of the information provided to airport passengers and staff in meeting their information needs.

The leading question was: what does the public want to know – and are knowledge and information adapted into behaviour?

The collection of empirical data took place on the third day (April 29, 2009) of public health measures at the airport and concerns the very early stage of the management of a pandemic, which may have implications for how we react to future outbreaks and evolving pandemics.

---

[2] According to the EU Law and the International Health Regulations (IHR) the primary security line means the physical set of barriers of the airport that separate the unrestricted landside area from the restricted airside area

This study was published in the journal *Influenza and Other Respiratory Viruses* (Dickmann, Petra and Rubin, G. James and Gaber, Walter and Wicker, Sabine and Wessely, Simon and Serve, Hubert and Gottschalk, René (2011) *New Influenza A/H1N1 ("Swine Flu"): information needs of airport passengers and staff*. Influenza and other respiratory viruses, 5 (1). 39-46).

Common Perspective

The two studies present two sides of the same coin, while the first relates to more extreme behavioural reactions among unexposed members of the public (seeking healthcare) and is necessarily literature-based given that it was conducted prior to the pandemic, the second is based on lower levels of concern that can still have an impact on behaviours such as reporting of symptoms.

The leading question of the first part was: what is known and what data is available about information needs and predictors of behavioural response to infectious disease? The second part though provides data about the information needs, describes the evolving situation and concludes with recommendations for risk and crisis communication strategies.

Both parts follow their own structure regarding format, quotation style and literature which was due to meet the requirements of the respective journal.

How to Reduce the Impact of 'Low Risk Patients' following a Bioterrorist Incident: Lessons Learned from SARS, Anthrax and Pneumonic Plague

G. James Rubin[1] & Petra Dickmann[2,3]

1) King's College London, UK
2) Johann Wolfgang Goethe-University Frankfurt am Main, Germany
3) Humboldt University Berlin, Germany

Investigation Period: March 2008 – October 2008
Report for the British Home Office: October 2008
Submitted at the journal *Biosecurity and Bioterrorism*. April 2009
Accepted with reviewer comments: Juni 2009
Resubmitted final version: November 2009
Accepted: December 15, 2009
Publication Date: March 2010

G James Rubin and Petra Dickmann (2010): *How to Reduce the Impact of "Low Risk Patients" following a Bioterrorist Incident: Lessons Learned form SARS, Anthrax and Pneumonic Plague*, Biosecurity and Bioterrorism, March 2010, 8(1), 37-43.

Reprint with kind permission from Mary Ann Liebert, Inc. publishers

Abstract

A bioterrorist attack may result in a large number of unexposed patients attending medical facilities in search of treatment or reassurance. In this paper, we review evidence from three previous biological incidents that are analogous to a bioterrorist attack in order to gauge the likely incidence of such 'low risk patients' and to identify possible strategies for coping with this phenomenon. Evidence from the anthrax attacks in the United States suggested that a surge of low risk patients is by no means inevitable. Data from the SARS outbreak illustrated that if hospitals are seen as sources of contagion, many patients with non-bioterrorism related health care needs may delay seeking help. Finally, the events surrounding the pneumonic plague outbreak of 1994 in Surat, India, highlighted the need for the public to be kept adequately informed about an incident. Although it is impossible to say what the likely incidence of low risk patients will be during a future bioterrorist incident, several strategies may help to reduce it and to safeguard the well-being of the low risk patients themselves. These include the provision of clear information about who should and should not attend hospital, the use of telephone services to provide more detailed information and initial screening, rapid triage at hospital entrances based where possible on exposure history and objective signs of illness, and subsequent telephone follow-up of those judged to be at low risk. (232 words)

Introduction

Bioterrorism has the potential to place great strain on a region's medical services. While patients requiring emergency care may represent a substantial caseload, a greater issue may be the accompanying influx of unexposed patients who wish to be assessed, decontaminated and treated. Many of these patients may report physical symptoms that can be hard to differentiate from the symptoms of exposure to a bioterrorist agent, but which have their origin in psychological mechanisms or are the result of other conditions that are unrelated to the attack[1;2]. Other patients may attend hospital with acute psychological distress, due to exacerbation of a psychiatric disorder, or because they wish to obtain more information about the incident. Finding an appropriate term for this heterogeneous group is difficult. The phrase 'worried well' which is sometimes used is now seen as disparaging, inaccurate and unhelpful and should no longer be applied. A better term may be "low risk patient"[3]. While identifying which individual patients are genuinely at low risk may present difficulties in some incidents, particularly those where exposure status is difficult to confirm, for other incidents the term is easier to apply. The phrase also allows for a degree of uncertainty about risk status and has reassuring connotations for the patient.

The arrival of large numbers of low risk patients at hospitals following bioterrorism would be problematic for three main reasons[3-5]. First, it would complicate the situation at hospitals receiving exposed patients, delaying the treatment of the acutely ill, creating difficulties of crowd control and tying up medical resources. Second, for the low risk patients themselves, attending hospital following a bioterrorist attack might increase their risk of exposure to the agent in question, as well as their risk of misdiagnoses and inappropriate treatment. Third, the needs of low risk patients may be poorly attended to at hospitals which are already overstretched dealing with medical casualties. Although not direct victims of the attack per se, many low risk patients nonetheless have genuine healthcare needs and require suitable reassurance. If inappropriately handled, the potential exists for the physical symptoms and distress experienced by some of these patients to become chronic problems[2].

Although concern exists about the likelihood of a surge of low risk patients affecting hospitals and other health care resources following bioterrorism, little is known about the characteristics of such a phenomenon or the possible interventions that might ameliorate it. In this report, we review the incidence and impact of low risk patients in relation to three previous infectious disease incidents; the anthrax attacks in the USA during 2001, the outbreak of severe acute respiratory syndrome (SARS) in 2002 and 2003, and the outbreak of pneumonic plague in Surat in 1994. These outbreaks were chosen because they represent a genuine bioterrorist attack (anthrax[6]), a natural outbreak of a potential bioterrorism agent which at the time was widely rumoured to be a deliberate release (pneumonic plague[7]) and a major outbreak of a novel emerging pathogen which required some hospitals to activate their bioterrorism protocols in order to cope with the incident (SARS[8]). Data relating to these incidents are used to characterise likely low risk patient behaviours and to suggest possible strategies for dealing with them.

Methods

A search of Medline allowed us to identify publications that might contain relevant data (search strategy available on request). For the anthrax and SARS outbreaks, papers expressing only expert opinion or anecdotal evidence were excluded. However, given the paucity of relevant data for the pneumonic plague outbreak in Surat, such evidence was included where relevant for this incident.

Results

Anthrax

Impact on attendance at hospitals and other health care facilities

We identified one study which provided quantitative data on changing patterns of hospital usage during the time period of the US anthrax attacks[9]. According to this retrospective analysis for 15 New Jersey emergency departments, all within a 55 mile radius of one of the anthrax incidents, an increase in the number of patients whose notes indicated that they were "screened for infectious disease" but who had "no diagnosis of feared complaint" occurred immediately after the first local anthrax case was identified[9]. In absolute terms, however, this increase represented only 0.92% of all emergency department visits during that period, although for the two hospitals closest to the affected postal facility this figure doubled to 1.8%[9]. A second study, concerning one large primary care facility in New York, also noted a rise in patient visits following the attacks compared with either the previous or subsequent years[10]. However, out of all 30,456 contacts with patients that were recorded by the practice between 11 September and 21 December 2001, only 244 involved any patient-initiated discussion about bioterrorism (0.8%). Of the 241 individual patients involved, 97 reported potential exposure (either to a white powder or because of working in a mail room) and 110 reported subjective symptoms. Twenty-one percent requested antibiotics[10].

Surveys of the general public confirmed that there was a relatively low level of health care use among low risk individuals as a direct result of the anthrax attacks. Only 5% in one survey reported that they, or anyone else in their household, had spoken to a doctor about health issues relating to bioterrorism, while only 3% reported that they or someone else from the household had spoken to a health professional about their anxieties relating to the attacks[11]. These data do hide a degree of variability however: within areas involved in an incident, individuals who reported that they, a close friend or a family member had been caught up in the anthrax events were more likely to have spoken to a physician about anthrax-related concerns or anxiety, or to have obtained a prescription for antibiotics[11].

Demand for antibiotics

Evidence was found that some low risk US citizens requested, and received, prescriptions for ciprofloxacin and doxycycline (the two antibiotics recommended as primary prophylactic agents against anthrax). One assessment of prescriptions given out by pharmacies across the US noted large increases in the distribution of both drugs in October 2001 compared to October 2000, despite relative stability in prescriptions for other antibiotics, with prescribing of the two drugs increasing by roughly 160,000 and 96,000 courses, respectively[12]. This does not imply that these drugs were actually consumed, however; stockpiling by concerned members of the public may also explain the increase. For instance, general public surveys found that while 4% reported that they, or someone else in the household, had obtained a prescription for antibiotics, less than 0.5% had actually taken the medication[11]. This increased prescribing of antibiotics to low risk patients was also identified by others, using both prescribing trend data and surveys of physicians[10;13;14].

Impact on other health-care resources

During the attacks, telephone hotlines were set up to deal with calls from the public or healthcare professionals. These came under some pressure. One location received 25,000 such calls during a two week period, while nine other states recorded 2,817 calls during the course of a week[6]. During one month, the CDC Emergency Operations Centre logged 11,063 anthrax related calls, of which only 882 were referred to a second tier State Liaison Team[15]. Although most of these related to low risk patients, only 20% of these calls actually came from members of the public, with most coming from healthcare workers and state or federal employees. As such, the hotline does not seem to have been used primarily by people seeking reassurance for symptoms unrelated to exposure. Instead, the commonest reason for calling related to requests for general bioterrorism information[15]. As well as phoning call centres, US citizens also turned to the internet during the attacks to obtain more information[11], with use of the www.cdc.gov website increasing by 100%[16].

Severe Acute Respiratory Syndrome (SARS)
Overall impact on health-care resources
One key feature of the SARS outbreak was the high number of hospital acquired infections that occurred; of 8096 cases, 1706 (21%) occurred in health care workers[17]. This had a major impact on the number of patients attending hospital for any reason during the outbreak. Using a retrospective review of charts in one Taiwanese hospital assigned to accept SARS patients, Huang et al reported a 44% reduction in adult patients attending the emergency department during the peak of the outbreak[18]. This reduction occurred primarily in patients with a less urgent need to be seen; no change was found in the number of patients arriving by ambulance, with a critical or life threatening illness or requiring admission to a ward or to intensive care. Many other hospitals reported similar declines in non-SARS related visits[19-24], while data from Taiwan's National Health Insurance program showed significant declines in expenditure for both ambulatory and inpatient care during the period of the outbreak[25]. Further analysis of insurance data showed that reductions were particularly evident for respiratory diseases, minor problems and elective surgery, and less so for acute conditions, mental disorders or essential treatment that could not be postponed[26].

Why did hospitals witness such reductions in patient numbers? The periodic closure of services, public appeals for patients with minor illnesses to stay away and concern among some members of the public about possible detention if they were found to be febrile may all have contributed[19;21;23;27]. But given that declines in hospital attendance also tended to be linked to media reporting of SARS cases, that an increase in patients discharging themselves from hospital against medical advice was observed, and that the general public endorsed staying away from hospitals as a useful way of avoiding SARS, it seems probable that fear of acquiring SARS was a key reason for the reductions[21;24;28].

Importantly, though, while non-essential use of hospitals declined, this does not mean that patients no longer sought help for non-SARS related conditions. Instead, a shift in the way that help was sought was identified in several studies. For example, in Toronto, both

Telehealth Ontario (a 24 hour medical advice line) and primary care physicians reported a large increase in the number of consultations being given by phone[23]. Meanwhile analysis of health insurance data suggested that for certain conditions, smaller district hospitals and clinics (which were less willing or able to take SARS patients) also witnessed an increase in patient numbers[26;29].

Use of health-care resources by low risk patients

Although the most striking finding from the SARS outbreak was the overall fall in patient attendance at hospitals, of those who did attend many were low risk patients. For instance, Boutis et al. cited otherwise unpublished data from two Toronto hospitals[23]. One hospital reported screening "more than 1000 concerned members of the public, 70 of whom met the case definition of suspected or probable SARS." The other hospital reported that "up to 50% of presenting patients had concerns that their symptoms were SARS-related." More rigorous data were available from Singapore, where the main hospital responsible for treating SARS assessed 11,461 patients in a triage centre set up outside the main emergency department entrance[8]. This process involved checking for the presence of fever and administering a simple questionnaire to assess exposure history and symptoms. Of all patients screened in this way, only 1,386 (12%) were subsequently admitted to the hospital for further assessment[8]. Of the remaining 10,075, it subsequently transpired that 28 did have probable or suspected SARS and had been misclassified. The remainder (88%) were categorised as low risk, with the authors noting that "the majority were either asymptomatic or had minor ailments such as upper respiratory tract infection." These patients were provided with education about SARS, reassurance, and telephone follow-up over the next two weeks.

This experience was also mirrored in one Taiwanese hospital, which received requests for screening from 1,421 "individuals who had no documented fever or exposure history"[30]. These 1,421 low risk patients, many of whom reported various medically unexplained symptoms, accounted for 64% of all potential SARS patients who were seen[30].

As well as attending hospital, low risk patients also accessed other resources. In Taiwan, a dedicated SARS fever hotline was set up with the specific intention of triaging patients with fever and reducing the number of low risk patients attending hospital[31]. A separate telephone number for individuals seeking general information rather than medical advice was also provided. Within an 11 day period the fever hotline received 11,228 calls. Of these, 28%

were advised to seek medical assistance, 21% were advised to remain at home and monitor their symptoms, while the majority (51%) received general advice but did not require any specific medical recommendations. Of callers for whom data were available, only 37% actually had a fever.

Meanwhile, within Hong Kong, 5% of the public in one survey reported getting health information about SARS from medical professionals[28]. This contrasts with 19% of Toronto residents, and 6% of US residents[32]

Pneumonic Plague

On 19 September 1994 three patients with pneumonic plague were admitted to the New Civil Hospital in the Indian city of Surat, triggering a major public health response. In total, the incident eventually resulted in 56 deaths[33] and caused enormous public fear and a large-scale spontaneous surge of people away from the city. This was partly the result of ill-informed, inconsistent or incomplete information given out during the crises[34].

Perhaps the most notable low risk patient behaviour observed across India during this outbreak was the intensive and wide-spread purchasing of those medicines that were reported in the media to act as a prophylaxis against plague, including tetracycline and a homeopathic preparation called phosphorus 30[7;35-37]. This 'panic buying' placed pressure on stocks of these medications[34;35;38]. In addition, it was widely recognised at the time that many patients arriving at hospital for assessment did not have plague[39]. Partly this problem stemmed from poor case-definitions and limited triage arrangements. As news reports noted "the standard response [from physicians around India] has been to admit patients with 'plague-like symptoms' to hospital" with doctors "referring many patients with high fever, cough and chest pain to the hospitals reserved for cases of plague." Unfortunately, this loose definition also encompassed tuberculosis, pneumonia and malaria[39]. In addition to misdiagnosis, self-referring low risk patients also contributed to the problem, with hospitals in Dehli becoming "flooded" with anxious patients[34] while the New Civil Hospital was reported as being "packed with plague and the worried well"[40]. As one expert later observed "a little runny nose and a cough, you were immediately rushed to the hospital"[34]. This phenomenon may go some way towards explaining the puzzled comments that some experts made regarding the outbreak: "Almost all the patients had mild illness. High fever was uncommon, and a significant number had no fever at all. The look of the affected persons failed to reveal that they were having a serious disease" [35].

Discussion

Estimates of the potential incidence of low risk patients following a future bioterrorist attack can vary widely[5]. In truth, however, it is impossible to give any firm estimate: while some previous examples have resulted in a large number of low risk patients seeking access to health care services, other examples such as the anthrax attacks have resulted in less health anxiety among the unexposed public. Several factors help to explain why the incidence can differ so dramatically. First, the perceived risk associated with the incident is clearly crucial, with factors which increase the dread or outrage felt by the public (e.g. Surat), or the perceived likelihood of being affected by the incident serving to moderate the likelihood of individuals utilizing health care resources. With regard to this latter point, the geographical or occupational restriction of any risk and also whether a disease is perceived to be contagious or not are clearly key factors to consider (e.g. Anthrax). Second, a population's perceptions about the nature of the agent involved and whether health care services can offer effective protection or treatment will also be important. This is true regardless of the validity of these perceptions: in Surat, for instance, the wide spread purchasing of tetracycline and phosphorus 30 was triggered by media reporting of their prophylactic powers, not by the objective efficacy of either drug[34]. Third, the perceived risk-benefit trade-off involved in attending health-care facilities will also determine how many low risk patients use them. Where hospitals are viewed as potential sources of contagion, as in SARS, this will restrict the attendance of low risk patients. Fourth, the availability of alternative resources which meet the needs of low risk patients will also be important. This can range from trusted organisations providing credible information about when to seek help, to resources specifically allocated to assessing, advising and reassuring low risk patients on a one-to-one basis[15;31]. Finally, even the definition of 'low risk patient' will differ across incidents, depending on the specific nature of the threat. For example, an overt release of infectious material that is identified early may differ from a covert release that goes undetected for some time in terms of how authorities must define 'high risk,' and hence 'low risk,' patients. In some circumstances, any patient reporting flu-like symptoms may need to be considered at risk, even if this will inevitably include some patients whose symptoms are attributable to other causes.

Strategies for reducing the impact of low risk patients

Our review suggests several strategies which may help to reduce the impact of low risk patients following bioterrorism. These largely concur with previous recommendations[3-5]. In the immediate aftermath of an attack, providing information as quickly as possible about who should seek medical attention, and who should not, will be essential[3]. Clear, consistent messages of this type helped keep patient numbers to manageable levels during the SARS outbreak[19;23]. In order to reduce attendance by patients with symptoms that are not attributable to the incident, such information should ideally specify objective criteria such as exposure or fever as the criteria for seeking help. Depending on the incident, however, this may not always be possible. Continually updated, credible information concerning the incident in general should also be provided. In previous incidents, a substantial motivation for low risk patients to interact with the health services has been their desire to obtain more information[10;11;15;31]. The use of a continually updated internet resource is one route that may help to provide this level of detailed information to concerned members of the public, while reducing the pressure on medical services.

Inevitably, however, some people will still wish to discuss their concerns with a clinician. If local regulations allow it, then facilities to provide remote, one-to-one advice and assessment away from hospitals must therefore also be in place, with telephone consultations remaining the most pragmatic way of providing this. Experience from the SARS and anthrax incidents suggest that telephone helplines providing general information and preliminary medical assessments were used by members of the public who might otherwise have presented at hospitals or primary care facilities[15;31].

Regardless of what preventive steps are taken, some low risk patients will nonetheless present at hospital or primary care practices. Rapid triage of patients, based wherever possible on exposure history or objective clinical signs will therefore be required to identify those requiring immediate treatment. While some authors have suggested that "low risk patient facilities" or "support centres" be used to house patients turned away from triage points, providing a venue in which to give out information and conduct further assessment[3-5], in the context of an infectious disease outbreak in which there is a risk of person to person transmission a better approach may be to ask patients to return home following triage and after the provision of information and reassurance, with the promise that further follow-up by telephone will occur[8]. This would help to reduce the risk of contagion, allow a patient's psychological state to be assessed over a lengthier time-course, reassure patients that they have not been forgotten and provide a secondary stage of triage, allowing patients who were initially miscategorised to be identified and recalled to hospital[8].

Reductions in the use of medical services during an incident.

While unnecessary use of health care resources by low risk patients is of concern, our review also suggested that consideration be given to patients who require medical help for conditions unrelated to an attack but who will either delay seeking help or change the way in which they access health care services through fear of coming into contact with the bioterrorist threat. This is particularly likely to be the case for infectious diseases with high rates of person to person transmission. This phenomenon, observed most clearly in the SARS outbreak, can result in dramatic declines in patient numbers at major hospitals, together with increased use of smaller facilities and telephone consultations[23]. While explicitly demonstrating to patients that hospitals remain safe to visit may help to reduce this effect, planners should be aware that telephone-based healthcare resources and smaller health-care facilities may require additional resources to cope with increased demand following bioterrorism.

Conclusions

Our review highlighted several key lessons that could be learned from the SARS, anthrax and pneumonic plague incidents which may help in preparing for the challenges presented by low risk patients following a future terrorist attack. In particular, we have noted several features of an incident that may have a large impact on the nature and magnitude of changes in behaviour in the unexposed population, we have highlighted the need to plan for decreased use of hospitals following a major incident and we have suggested the need for adequate telephone facilities to allow low-risk patients to access information, early triage and subsequent follow-up, as required.

We would, however, also raise one important caveat. The scientific literature on low risk patient behaviour following major incidents is sparse, particularly with regards to good quality data concerning the incidence, motivations or outcomes of low risk patients, or the efficacy of different strategies for reducing their impact on the health care services and for ensuring that their own well-being is looked after[3]. Many of the suggestions contained within this paper are thus speculative. A need exists for more research into each of these issues, beginning with a prospective cohort study of all patients who present at health care facilities following the next major chemical, biological or radiological incident.

Acknowledgements

This review was funded by the UK Home Office. James Rubin worked on the review under the terms of Career Development research training Fellowship issued by the UK National Institute for Health Research. Petra Dickmann is a visiting research associate who worked on the review as part of her medical dissertation. The views expressed in this publication are those of the authors and not necessarily those of the NHS, the NIHR, the UK Department of Health or the Home Office.

Reference List

(1) Page LA, Petrie KJ, Wessely S. Psychosocial responses to environmental incidents: A review and a proposed typology. J Psychosom Res 2006; 60:413-422.

(2) Hyams KC, Murphy FM, Wessely S. Responding to chemical, biological or nuclear terrorism: the indirect and long-term health effects may present the greatest challenge. J Health Polit Policy Law 2002; 27(2):273-291.

(3) Stone FP. The "Worried Well" Response to CBRN Events: Analysis and Solutions. Alabama: USAF Counterproliferation Center; 2007.

(4) Shultz JM, Espinel Z, Galea S, Shaw JA, Miller GT. Surge, Sort, Support: Disaster behavioral health for health care professionals. Miami: Disaster Epidemiology Emergency Preparedness Centre; 2006.

(5) Engel CC, Locke S, Reissman DB, DeMartino R, Kutz I, McDonald M et al. Terrorism, trauma and mass casualty triage: How might we solve the latest mind-body problem? Biosecurity and Bioterrorism: Biodefense Strategy, Practice, and Science 2007; 5(2):155-163.

(6) United States General Accounting Office. Bioterrorism: Public Health Response to Anthrax Incidents of 2001. Washington DC: US GAO; 2003.

(7) Raza G, Dutt B, Singh S. Kaleidoscoping public understanding of science on hygiene, health and plague: a survey in the aftermath of a plague epidemic in India. Public Understanding of Science 1997; 6:247-267.

(8) Tham K-Y. An emergency department response to severe acute respiratory syndrome: A prototype response to bioterrorism. Ann Emerg Med 2004; 43(1):6-14.

(9) Allegra PC, Cochrane D, Dunn E, Milano P, Rothman J, Allegra J. Emergency department visits for concern regarding anthrax - New Jersey, 2001. MMWR 2005; 54 (supplement):163-167.

(10) Hupert N, Chege W, Bearman GML, Pelzman FN. Antibiotics for anthrax; patient requests and physician prescribing practices during the 2001 New York City attacks. Arch Intern Med 2004; 164:2012-2016.

(11) Blendon RJ, Benson JM, DesRoches CM, Pollard WE, Parvanta C, Hermann MJ. The impact of anthrax attacks on the American public. Medscape General Medicine 2002; 4(2).

(12) Shaffer D, Armstrong G, Higgins K, Honig P, Coyne P, Boxwell D et al. Increased US prescription trends associated with the CDC Bacillus anthracis antimicrobial postexposure prophylaxis campaign. Pharacomepidemiology and Drug Safety 2003; 12:177-182.

(13) Brinker A, Pamer C, Beitz J. Changes in Ciprofloxacin Utilization as Shown in a Large Pharmacy Claims Database: Effects of Proximity to Criminal Anthrax Exposure in October 2001. J Am Pharm Assoc (Wash) 2003; 43:375-378.

(14) M'ikanatha NM, Julian KG, Kunselman AR, Aber RC, Rankin JT, Lautenbach E. Patients' request for and emergency physicians' prescription of antimicrobial prophylaxis for anthrax during the 2001 bioterrorism-related outbreak. BMC Public Health 2005; 5(2).

(15) Mott JA, Treadwell TA, Hennessy TW, Rosenberg PA, Wolfe MI, Brown CM et al. Call tracking data and the public health response to bioterrorism-related anthrax. Emerg Infect Dis 2002; 8(10):1088-1092.

(16) Hobbs J, Kittler A, Fox S, Middleton B, Bates DW. Communicating health information to an alarmed public facing a threat such as bioterrorism. Journal of Health Communication 2004; 9:67-75.

(17) World Health Organisation. Summary of probable SARS cases with onset of illness from 1 November 2002 to 31 July 2003. http://www.who.int/csr/sars/country/table2004_04_21/en/print.html: WHO; 2003.

(18) Huang C-C, Yen DHT, Huang H-H, Kao W-F, Wang L-M, Huang C-I et al. Impact of severe acute respiratory syndrome (SARS) outbreaks on the use of emergency department medical resources. 68 2005; 6(254):259.

(19) Tsai MC, Arnold JL, Chuang CC, Chi CH, Liu CC, Yang YJ. Impact of an outbreak of severe acute respiratory syndrome on a hospital in Taiwan, ROC. Emergency Medicine Journal 2004; 21:311-316.

(20) Chen Y-C, Chen M-F, Liu S-Z, Romeis JC, Lee Y-T. SARS in teaching hospital, Taiwan. Emerg Infect Dis 2004; 10(10):1886-1887.

(21) Man CY, Yeung RSD, Chung JYM, Cameron PA. The impact of SARS on an emergency department in Hong Kong. Emerg Med 2003; 15:418-422.

(22) Chen T-A, Lai K-H, Chang H-T. Impact of a severe acute respiratory syndrome outbreak in the emergency department: an experience in Taiwan. Emergency Medicine Journal 2003; 21:660-662.

(23) Boutis K, Stephens D, Lam K, Ungar WJ, Schuh S. The impact of SARS on a tertiary care pediatric emergency department. CMAJ 2004; 171(11):1353-1358.

(24) Heiber M, Lou WYW. Effect of the SARS outbreak on visits to a community hospital emergency department. Canadian Journal of Emergency Medicine 2006; 8(5):323-328.

(25) Chang HJ, Huang N, Lee C-H, Hsu Y-J, Hsieh C-J, Chou Y-J. The impact of the SARS epidemic on the utilization of medical services: SARS and the fear of SARS. Am J Public Health 2004; 94(4):562-564.

(26) Lu T-H, Chou Y-J, Liou C-S. Impact of SARS on healthcare utilization by disease categories: Implications for delivery of healthcare services. Health Policy 2007; 83:375-381.

(27) Haines CJ, Chu TKH, Chung TKH. The effect of Severe Acute Respiratory Syndrome on a hospital obstetrics and gynaecology service. Br J Obstet Gynaecol 2003; 110:643-645.

(28) Lau JTF, Yang X, Tsui H, Kim JH. Monitoring community responses to the SARS epidemic in Hong Kong: from day 10 to day 62. J Epidemiol Community Health 2003; 57:864-870.

(29) Lee C-H, Huang N, Chang H-J, Hsu Y-J, Wang M-C, Chou Y-J. The immediate effects of the severe acute respiratory syndrome (SARS) epidemic on childbirth in Taiwan. BMC Public Health 2005; 5:30.

(30) Chen S-Y, Ma MHM, Su C-P, Chiang W-C, Ko PCI, Lai T-I. Facing an outbreak of highly transmissible disease: Problems in emergency department response. Ann Emerg Med 2004; 44:93-95.

(31) Kaydos-Daniels SC, Olowokure B, Chang H-J, Barwick RS, Deng J-F, Lee M-L et al. Body temperature monitoring and SARS fever hotline, Taiwan. Emerg Infect Dis 2004; 10(2):373-376.

(32) Blendon RJ, Benson JM, DesRoches CM, Raleigh E, Taylor-Clark K. The public's response to the severe acute respiratory syndrome in Toronto and the United States. Clin Infect Dis 2004; 38:925-931.

(33) CDC. Update: human plague - India, 1994. Morbidity and Mortality Weekly Report 2008; 43:761-762.

(34) Ramalingaswami V. Psychological effects of the 1994 plague outbreak in Surat, India. Mil Med 2001; 166:29.

(35) Deodhar NS, Yemul VL, Banerjee K. Plague that never was: A review of the alleged plague outbreaks in India in 1994. J Public Health Policy 1998; 19:184-199.

(36) Nandan G. Troops battle to contain India's outbreak of plague. BMJ 1994.

(37) Mavalankar DV. Plague in India. Lancet 1994; 344:1298.

(38) Madan TN. The plague in India, 1994. Soc Sci Med 1995; 40(9):1167-1168.

(39) Nandan G. Plague spreads in India but is "under control". BMJ 1994; 309:897.

(40) Garrett L. Betrayal of Trust: The Collapse of Global Public Health. Oxford: Oxford University Press; 2001.

APPENDIX A

Search Strategy

Database: Ovid MEDLINE(R) <1950 to April Week 2 2008>

Search Strategy:

----

1   exp Attitude to Health/ or exp Health Services Misuse/ or exp "Patient Acceptance of Health Care"/ or exp Managed Care Programs/ or exp Somatoform Disorders/ or exp Anxiety/ or worried well.mp. or exp Health Education/

2   exp Questionnaires/ or exp Needs Assessment/ or exp "Health Services Needs and Demand"/ or exp Information Systems/ or exp Health Education/ or exp Patient Education as Topic/ or exp Information Services/ or Information Need.mp.

3   exp Health Knowledge, Attitudes, Practice/ or exp Risk Assessment/ or exp Communication/ or risk communication.mp. or exp Risk/

4   exp Emergency Service, Hospital/ or hospital attendance.mp.

5   health care.mp. or exp "Delivery of Health Care"/

6   1 or 2 or 3 or 4 or 5

7   **exp Anthrax/ or anthrax.mp.**

8   **6 and 7**

****

SEARCHES 7 AND 8

These searches were adjusted depending on the specific outbreak.

New Influenza A/H1N1 ("Swine Flu"): Information Needs of Airport Passengers and Staff

Petra Dickmann[1,2], G. James Rubin[3], Walter Gaber[4], Simon Wessely[3], Sabine Wicker[1], Hubert Serve[1], Rene Gottschalk[1,5]

1) Johann Wolfgang Goethe-University Frankfurt am Main, Germany (P. Dickmann, S. Wicker, H. Serve, R. Gottschalk)

2) Humboldt University Berlin, Germany (P. Dickmann)

3) King's College London, UK (G.J. Rubin, S. Wessely)

4) Fraport AG, Frankfurt am Main, Germany (W. Gaber)

5) Health Protection Authority, City of Frankfurt am Main, Germany (R. Gottschalk)

published:

Dickmann, Petra and Rubin, G. James and Gaber, Walter and Wicker, Sabine and Wessely, Simon and Serve, Hubert and Gottschalk, René (2011) *New Influenza A/H1N1 ("Swine Flu"): information needs of airport passengers and staff.* Influenza and other respiratory viruses, 5 (1), 39-46.

Reprint with kind permission from John Wiley and Sons

Abstract

Airports are the entrances of infectious diseases. Particularly at the beginning of an outbreak information and communication play an important role to enable the early detection of signs or symptoms and to encourage passengers to adopt appropriate preventive behaviour in order to limit the spread of the disease.

At the start of the Influenza A/H1N1 epidemic (April 29-30, 2009) qualitative semi structured interviews (N=101) were conducted at Frankfurt International Airport with passengers who were either returning from or going to Mexico and with airport staff who had close contact with these passengers. Interviews focused on knowledge about swine flu, information needs and anxiety concerning the outbreak. The aim of the study was to determine the adequacy of the information provided to airport passengers and staff in meeting their information needs. The results showed that perceived information needs were directly related to anxiety – the least anxious participants did not want any additional information, while the most anxious participants reported a range of information needs. Information needs were the same irrespective of actual or potential exposure. Airport staff in contact with passengers travelling from the epicentre of the outbreak showed the highest levels of anxiety, coupled with a desire to be adequately briefed by their employer.

Our results suggest that information strategies should address not only the exposed or potentially exposed but also groups that feel at risk; further communication strategies based on information about the disease and advice about effective preventive behaviours may be particularly useful in the management of infectious diseases. (251 words)

Introduction

Airports are common entrances of infectious diseases and air travel has become the most effective transmission route for emerging infectious diseases. Some infectious diseases are manageable at the airport with conventional medical screenings like temperature screening (Gaber et al. 2009) because patients are only contagious after they show symptoms (e.g. SARS; Bell 2004). Other infectious diseases like influenza require special screening efforts, because patients may transmit the disease before they show symptoms. Therefore, early detection of suspect cases was one priority of public health measures at the beginning of the swine flu outbreak. One major strategy was to inform airport passengers about the early signs and symptoms of the disease and to communicate advice how to behave, if they suspect themselves to suffer from the disease. It was the hope that this could enable and encourage travellers to protect themselves and to prevent the spread of infection. Various studies have assessed information needs and behavioural changes among the general public in response to the swine flu outbreak (e.g. Rubin et al. 2009, Seale et al. 2009, Quinn et al. 2009). However, airport passengers and staff represent groups of particular interest, given their high potential to spread the disease. Illness in these populations must be detected quickly and adequate preventive behaviour has to be effectively encouraged. Promoting awareness of the nature of swine flu among these groups may help to ensure that people with symptoms consistent with swine flu make themselves known to public health officials and should provide useful information about preventive behaviour including strict hygiene.

This is research about what happened during the earliest stages of the 2009 swine flu pandemic, which may have implications for how we react to future outbreaks and evolving pandemics (Fraser et al. 2009). Our main assumptions were that obtaining early information about symptoms, isolating infected patients and communicating behaviour advice that includes practising strict hygiene is the most effective strategy to interrupt the chain of infection among members of the public in the absence of specific prophylaxis (Barry 2009, Funk et al. 2009, Glik 2007).

Public health measures at the airport

In Germany, public health measures relating to airline travel began on Monday, April 27, 2009 with on-board screening of, and information provision to, passengers on flights coming from Mexico. Roughly 460 passengers per day arrived on direct flights from Mexico and were seen by two doctors, one from the airport and one from the health authorities, who provided information on board shortly after the plane landed. They also asked for passengers who were not feeling well to make themselves known. The detection of ill passengers was based on voluntary notice by sick passengers themselves or by appraisal of the doctors. Between 27 April and 30 April a leaflet (the 'airline leaflet') was given out to passengers at Frankfurt airport in three languages (German, English, Spanish). It contained health information for travellers coming from affected regions and was designed to raise awareness of the symptoms of swine flu and to encourage passengers to contact the flight crew if they had these symptoms or to consult a physician if they developed the symptoms within the next 7 days. The leaflet was based on information given by the German National public health institute (the Robert Koch-Institute), the local health authorities and the airport authorities (see Additional Material: Passenger leaflet). Other international airports distributed their own leaflets; therefore, passengers arriving at Frankfurt had various levels of knowledge and information.

Starting on April 27, airport staff was provided with a different leaflet and a document ("reading file") containing information about the disease and its transmissibility. Staff also received a workplace risk assessment which advised against the need for any protective equipment. This information highlighted the symptoms of swine flu and advised employees to contact a physician if they felt ill after close contact with a symptomatic passenger (see Additional Material: Staff leaflet).

Aim of the study

Future outbreaks of emerging infectious diseases are likely to follow a similar pattern with rapid spread of the disease through airline travel. We assume that an important measure against the spread is to insure knowledge about effective prevention and about the nature of the disease. Here, we report the results of qualitative semi structured interviews conducted at the beginning of the swine flu outbreak. These interviews were conducted at Frankfurt International Airport, one of the world's major air travel hubs. Interviews were conducted with passengers who were either returning from or going to Mexico, the country most affected by swine flu at the time, and with airport staff who had close contact with these passengers. Participants were assessed with respect to their knowledge, information needs and fears concerning the pandemic. Our aim was to determine the adequacy of the information provided to passengers and staff in terms of meeting their needs and enabling them to adapt their behaviours.

Methods

The study consisted of a series of semi-structured interviews conducted with passengers and members of staff at Frankfurt airport. Due to time constraints, a convenience sampling method was used, with participants approached as they waited for their bags, queued, or were arriving at their airport.

Procedure

Interviews were conducted on 29 and 30 April within Frankfurt airport. They were conducted in the secure areas at the gate, the international bus arrival and baggage reclaim. We interviewed passengers coming from Cancun and Mexico City and passengers going to Mexico City. The sample frame included all inbound and outbound flights between Frankfurt and Mexico during the period with a total of 1,418 passengers [Personal Communication from the Airline]. The interviews were conducted by one interviewer and took around 5 minutes to complete. Interviews were held in either German or English.

Participants

All passengers (age 14 upwards) who were travelling to or from Mexico were eligible for inclusion in the study. A smaller number of interviews were also carried out with airport staff who had close contact with passengers coming from affected regions. These included baggage claim personnel who assist travellers with enquiries about lost baggage and special care service employees who look after passengers with special needs in the terminal. We also interviewed customs officers who are often required to have body contact with passengers while screening for contraband.

We developed an interview guide for use with passengers, which contained 5 questions concerning information needs and fear levels (additional material 1). A similar 8-item interview guide was used with airport staff (additional material 2). For passengers, interview questions focused on departure and final destination; what information they had received about swine flu; what, if any, information needs they still had; and their current level of fear about swine flu on a scale of 0 (least fear) to 4 (most fear). For staff, the questions focused on their work routine; when they first heard about swine flu; when they were provided with information by the employer; what further information needs and wishes they had; and how they would classify their current fear level on a scale of 0 to 4.

Analysis

Fear scores were categorised as "0" no fear; "1-2" moderate fear; and "3-4" high fear. For statistical analyses contingency tables were performed as well as Chi-square tests for trend; where appropriate the Fisher's exact test was used. For the comparison of fear levels the Kruskal-Wallis-test was performed. Responses to open-ended questions were written down by the interviewer and subsequently categorized into the semantic answer.

Results

Participants

Of a total of 1,418 passengers (airline information) we approached 91 passengers (6.4%) to take part in the interview; 88 (97%) agreed to be interviewed. Of the staff groups we interviewed 100% (5/5) of the customs officers responsible on April, 29 for returning passengers from Mexico; 100% of special care service staff of the day shift on day one (2/2) and 50% on day two (1/2); and 50% (5/10) of the baggage claim day shift staff on day one. All staff groups in close contact with the returning passengers are represented in the sample. The demographic characteristics of both groups (travellers and staff) are given in table 1; the final destinations of the participants are given in table 2.

The information status of passengers

Only 19 of 50 (38%) inbound passengers had received the airline leaflet. We have no information why only 38% received information at the departing airport in Mexico. However, for those who had received it, it was their main information source. The information distribution at Mexico City Airport was described by passengers as poor. 12 passengers said they had received no information at all at the airport. Despite this, 35 of 50 (70%) felt sufficiently informed, primarily because of external information sources, for example the tour operator information service (mentioned by 13 participants), information from the media (mentioned by 19 participants) and information given by the doctors in Frankfurt on every plane from Mexico who checked the passengers at arrival. For outbound passengers, 26 of 38 (68%) had received the airline information leaflet. Four participants told us that they had consulted their GP before departure and travelled with Oseltamivir, masks and other protective equipment in their luggage. Consulting a GP was only reported on the second day of our investigation, possibly as a result of increased public alertness.

The information needs of passengers

35 of the 50 (70%) inbound travellers reported no further information needs. Those who had further information needs wanted to gather more information about medical (symptoms) and organisational ("what to do if I develop symptoms") issues. Of the outbound passengers travelling to Mexico only 12 of 38 (32%) had no further information needs. Most requested more information about protective behaviour (mentioned by 14 participants), the management of disease (8 participants), precise information about ongoing situation (6/38; 16%), contact details for health care services (5 participants) and the impact on daily life and future public health restriction (4 participants).

Fear level and information needs for passengers

The fear level for outbound passengers was significantly higher than for inbound passengers ($p<0.05$). In addition outbound passengers had substantially more information needs ($p<0.001$) compared to inbound passengers (table 3; figure 1). There was a highly significant relationship between fear level and information needs ($p<0.001$). Passengers who had a high fear level typically reported continuing information needs whereas passengers with a low or moderate fear level reported that they had sufficient information (table 3). This relationship was not affected by gender. Qualitative analysis of the data suggested that fear level and whether participants were inbound or outbound impacted on information needs. Inbound passengers with high anxiety reported needing more information about the recognition of relevant symptoms and a general awareness of contracting the disease. Outbound passengers with high anxiety needed more information about symptoms and medical advice.

Perception of public health measures among passengers

Arriving passengers had a generally positive perception of the public health measures adopted by the airport authorities. Even though we did not specifically ask about it, 13 of 50 (26%) respondents spontaneously gave positive feedback about the doctors on their plane as good communicators and as a primary source of information. Only 3 of 50 (6%) were critical about the public health measures, saying that the doctors screened people too quickly.

Further wishes of passengers

The additional comments made by inbound passengers included suggestions that they would appreciate a website by the airport offering relevant information about the situation and public health measures which arriving travellers could expect to encounter. Outbound passengers wished to have more protection equipment provided (masks) and needed more security advice for their trips.

Information status of staff

All employees had heard about swine flu over the weekend (25./26.04.09) in the media; in addition, two were phoned by colleagues over the weekend to inform them about the swine flu situation at the airport. Although they were exposed to returning passengers from the beginning of the outbreak, employees received their first official information from their employer relatively late: only two received a reading file on Monday (27.04.09), two received an email, two received a leaflet on Tuesday (28.04.09), three reported that they received information only after their own request on Wednesday (29.04.09) and one read information on the intranet on Wednesday (29.04.09). Three employees reported that they had received no information at all from the employer. Despite the worrying news from the media the employer's message was that there was no need to worry, because planes were assessed by the public health to be 'clean'. That this assessment was incorrect became obvious after the first infection among airport staff occurred in Germany.

Information needs of staff

Eleven employees had further information needs: about the protection measures, about symptoms and treatment and about their employer's policy regarding staff protection. The main communication problem identified was the recommendation by the employer that they should not wear masks even when in close contact with passengers from affected regions. This recommendation caused concern and misunderstanding, particularly because many of the passengers the staff were in contact with were wearing masks.

Further wishes of staff

The airport staff reported a desire to have a better medical and organizational briefing by a 'real' person and not just through leaflets or a reading file (mentioned by 11 participants). They felt at risk as first responders and needed not only information, but also attention and care from their employer. Most of them requested more practical advice for personal protection behaviour because the usual recommendation - keep your distance and wash hands frequently – did not seem feasible for their work place. All felt the need for an understanding by their employer for their work in terms of care, attention and acknowledgement.

Fear level of staff

The fear levels of the airport staff were very high (table 3) - which can be understood as a result of poor information level mixed with the difficult message about the corporate protection policy (no masks).

Discussion

Relation between anxiety and information needs

Our data suggested that a close relationship exists between anxiety and information needs: passengers and airport staff with a high fear level also had a poor information level. While we cannot be certain about the direction of causality implied by this association a parsimonious conclusion is that better information would assist in reducing anxiety in this population (Bowler 1994).

Further we conclude that inbound and outbound passengers as well as airport staff have relevant but different information needs: while inbound passengers wanted information about the management of the disease and medical and organisation procedures, outbound passengers needed to know more about protective behaviour, the evolving situation and contact details should they develop symptoms. Airport staff needed more information about the infectivity of the disease and appropriate protective behaviour in their work place. Tailored information for inbound and outbound passengers and for staff could meet these different needs. For the different fear levels of outbound passengers we observed that the information needs differed according to the fear level: low fear level participants needed information about *protective behaviour*; moderate fear participants needed information about *symptoms*; high fear participants needed both: protective behaviour *and* symptoms. This finding may have implications for future risk communication policy.

Information, Exposure and Fear Level

We found no significant relation between fear level and actual or potential exposure. Lack of information was associated with anxiety, irrespective of exposure. Focussing on actual exposure alone is not sufficient to meet information needs and/or reduce anxiety. As such any communication policy aimed solely at those exposed will be incomplete. Risk perception was more closely linked to emotional response and need for information than actual exposure. Thus the finding that those who were potentially exposed but reported adequate levels of information were not particularly anxious, whilst airport staff who felt potentially exposed but reported a lack of information were indeed anxious. This emphasises the importance of providing relevant information to airport staff as quickly as possible during an infectious diseases outbreak.

The association between poor information, uncertainty and anxiety has been noted several times before in the literature (Slovic 1987, Sandman 2009). Particularly for incidents where the health threat comes from a novel pathogen or chemical, uncertainty about the threat, conflicting messages from experts and the media, and confusing terminology or jargon can all result in increased levels of fear among the public (Speckhard 2002). Reducing uncertainty through the provision of clear information is therefore seen as important in its own right (Vyner 1988). A transparent information policy could help to reduce anxiety and irrational behaviour (Ofri 2009). Infection control measures rely mostly on individual behaviour, with effective communication enabling people to adopt that behaviour. This should be reflected in the future risk communication policy.

Perception of Public Health Measures: Personal Briefing

Doctors who checked the arriving passengers from Mexico in the inbound planes were seen as an appreciated, authentic and trustable source of information and participants welcomed their offer to address questions. The same is reported from the airport staff who stressed their need to have a 'real person' to inform, explain and answer questions (cf Rubin et al. 2007).

Relevance of Information

The relevance of timely and precise information is highly valuable in the management of infectious diseases (Jones & Salathe 2009). Information can reduce anxiety and enable public to behave appropriately to the evolving situation. Information and communication networks are the most effective instruments in the management of global outbreak while a prophylaxis or a specific pharmaceutical treatment is not yet available (Funk et al. 2009). Using the metaphor of the generic and specific human immune system, communication is the generic protection in the defensive process while prophylaxis and pharmaceutical treatment is the specific and adapted protection mechanism, which comes at a later stage.

Methodological limitations

Spreading outbreaks of potentially life threatening diseases can have an enormous effect on global economy, social life and health security (Gottschalk & Preiser 2005, Chang et al. 2004). Government and health protection authorities have a legitimate and pressing duty to prevent the import of swine flu cases, where possible. Assessing the impact of such measures needs to be done swiftly – hence we started this study within two days of the onset of the crisis in Germany. However, this meant that the sample was opportunistic, and not all measures equally validated. Data collection was also only possible over a two day period, because of aviation security legislation limiting access to secure areas for non essential staff.

Several specific caveats should therefore be borne in mind when evaluating this study. First, our use of convenience sampling may have biased the sample, with only those travellers or members of staff who were particularly interested in the topic being included in the sample. It is possible that we over-estimated the true level of concern within the population.

Second, due to logistical reasons we were unable to conduct interviews in Spanish, meaning that we may have a particularly unrepresentative sample for travellers arriving from Mexico.

Third, given the open-ended nature of our questions, it is difficult to determine what the genuine frequency of the various issues that we identified were in our sample. Had we used direct questioning with specified response options, the frequencies that we obtained may have been different.

Fourth, the location of our interviews may also have created some artefacts in our results. As travellers had not yet left the airport by the time of their interview, it is possible that some would have obtained more information after our interviews were concluded. We may therefore have underestimated the effectiveness of the communication within the airport.

Nonetheless, the importance of identifying key perceptions and communication difficulties during the very early stages of the swine flu outbreak outweighs these concerns. Had we delayed data collection by even a matter of days, public perceptions relating to swine flu would have been quantitatively and qualitatively different (Jones & Salathe 2009)

Conclusions

Airports are likely to be at the frontline of any future major infectious disease outbreak. Public health measures at a country's airports will play a large role in determining if and when a novel infectious disease enters the country. Providing information to inbound and outbound passengers, and to airport staff, should be seen as an integral part of these measures. This study has identified three ways in particular of maximising the effectiveness of this information. First, tailored information should be provided to these three groups, in order to tackle the different information priorities that they seem to have. Second, supplementing written information with an in-person briefing by a trusted source such as a doctor appears to be an effective way of reducing anxiety. This is particularly valuable if the communicator is able to take questions from the passengers and staff members. Third, information should include facts about symptoms of the disease and its incubation period, as well as advice on adequate preventive behaviour. The passenger leaflet only contained information about the symptoms of the disease and advice on what to do if the passenger experienced these symptoms. We consider it useful to include recommendations for the prevention and strict personal hygiene to limit the spread the disease.

Actual exposure risk is not the key determinant of public anxiety and desire for information, in contrast to the personal perception of being at risk. Risk communication strategies should address not only the exposed or potentially exposed but also the group that feels at risk in an appropriate and respectful way.

Our findings suggest ways to improve information provision in airports which plays a crucial role in the management of infectious diseases and pandemic outbreaks.

Future research is needed to design more effective communication strategies.

Ethics

This study was approved by the University Hospital of the JW Goethe-University Frankfurt am Main Ethics Commission (Reference number: 132/09).

Contribution of the authors

PD had the original idea for the study, devised the questionnaire, carried out the interviews and wrote the paper. GJR refined the questionnaire, advised on statistics and commented on the manuscript at all stages. WG assisted with the organisation of the study and commented on the manuscript. SW (London) assisted with the conception of the study, and rewrote the draft. SW (Frankfurt) and HS commented the statistics and the draft. RG did the statistics and tables and commented on the draft. He made the final approval of the version to be published and supervised the project.

All authors contributed extensively to the work presented in this paper

Conflict of Interests

None of the authors have a conflict of interest.

Financial support

There was no financial support for this research

References

Barry, J. M. (2009). Pandemics: avoiding the mistakes of 1918. *Nature, 459*(7245), 324-325.

Bell, D. M. (2004). Public health interventions and SARS spread, 2003. *Emerg Infect Dis, 10*(11), 1900-1906.

Bowler, R. M., Mergler, D., Huel, G., & Cone, J. E. (1994). Psychological, psychosocial, and psychophysiological sequelae in a community affected by a railroad chemical disaster. *J Trauma Stress, 7*(4), 601-624.

Chang, H. J., Huang, N., Lee, C. H., Hsu, Y. J., Hsieh, C. J., & Chou, Y. J. (2004). The impact of the SARS epidemic on the utilization of medical services: SARS and the fear of SARS. *Am J Public Health, 94*(4), 562-564.

Fraser, C., Donnelly, C. A., Cauchemez, S., Hanage, W. P., Van Kerkhove, M. D., Hollingsworth, T. D., et al. (2009). Pandemic potential of a strain of influenza A (H1N1): early findings. *Science, 324*(5934), 1557-1561.

Funk, S., Gilad, E., Watkins, C., & Jansen, V. A. (2009). The spread of awareness and its impact on epidemic outbreaks. *Proc Natl Acad Sci U S A, 106*(16), 6872-6877.

Gaber, W., Goetsch, U., Diel, R., Doerr, H. W., & Gottschalk, R. (2009). Screening for infectious diseases at international airports: the Frankfurt model. *Aviat Space Environ Med, 80*(7), 595-600.

Glik, D. C. (2007). Risk communication for public health emergencies. *Annu Rev Public Health, 28*, 33-54.

Gottschalk, R., & Preiser, W. (2005). Bioterrorism: is it a real threat? *Med Microbiol Immunol, 194*(3), 109-114.

Jones, J. H., & Salathe, M. (2009). Early assessment of anxiety and behavioral response to novel swine-origin influenza A(H1N1). *PLoS One, 4*(12), e8032.

Ofri, D. (2009). The Emotional Epidemiology of H1N1 Influenza Vaccination. *N Engl J Med*.

Quinn, S. C., Kumar, S., Freimuth, V. S., Kidwell, K., & Musa, D. (2009). Public willingness to take a vaccine or drug under Emergency Use Authorization during the 2009 H1N1 pandemic. *Biosecur Bioterror, 7*(3), 275-290.

Rubin, G. J., Amlot, R., Page, L., & Wessely, S. (2009). Public perceptions, anxiety, and behaviour change in relation to the swine flu outbreak: cross sectional telephone survey. *BMJ, 339*, b2651.

Rubin, G. J., Page, L., Morgan, O., Pinder, R. J., Riley, P., Hatch, S., et al. (2007). Public information needs after the poisoning of Alexander Litvinenko with polonium-210 in London: cross sectional telephone survey and qualitative analysis. *BMJ, 335*(7630), 1143.

Salkovskis, P. M., Rimes, K. A., Warwick, H. M., & Clark, D. M. (2002). The Health Anxiety Inventory: development and validation of scales for the measurement of health anxiety and hypochondriasis. *Psychol Med, 32*(5), 843-853.

Sandman, P. M. (2009). Pandemics: good hygiene is not enough. *Nature, 459*(7245), 322-323.

Seale, H., McLaws, M. L., Heywood, A. E., Ward, K. F., Lowbridge, C. P., Van, D., et al. (2009). The community's attitude towards swine flu and pandemic influenza. *Med J Aust, 191*(5), 267-269.

Slovic, P. (1987). Perception of risk. *Science, 236*(4799), 280-285.

Vyner, H. M. (1988). The psychological dimensions of health care for patients exposed to radiation and the other invisible environmental contaminants. *Soc Sci Med, 27*(10), 1097-1103.

APPENDIX B – ADDITIONAL MATERIAL

Passenger Questionnaire
Questions:
1. From what departure airport are you coming – and what is your destination?

2. Were you given any information about Swine flu at your departure airport? [YES or NO]

If yes "What did they tell you?"

3. What kind of information or advice would you find helpful at your destination?

4. On a scale of 0 to 4, where 0 is not at all and 4 is very much, how concerned are you about coming into contact with Swine Flu during your air travel today?

5. Can I ask which of these categories you fit into?
a) Men aged 18-30 (n=5)
b) Women aged 18-30 (n=5)
c) Men aged 31-60 (n=5)
d) Women aged 31-60 (n=5)
e) Men aged 61 plus (n=5)
f) Women aged 61 plus (n=5)

Airport staff
Questions
1. Place of work/duties
2. Working time overlapping with the beginning of disease (did you work over the weekend? Monday? Tuesday?)
3. When did first hear about swine flu? And where from (TV, newspaper, colleagues)?
4. When did your employer inform you about swine flu? What did he tell you/what can you remember?
5. Do you have further information needs from your employer?
6. If you could wish: what do you want your employer to do for you (behaviour of the employer question)?
7. On a scale from 0 (not at all) to 4 (very high): can you classify your fear of contracting the virus?
8. Male/female, age

Tables

Table 1: Basic data of participants

Passengers		Gender	No.	Total	Age
inbound		female	24		14-79
		male	26		26-61
	inbound Sum			50	14-79
outbound		female	17		14-69
		male	21		18-69
	outbound Sum			38	14-69
Subtotal				88	14-79
Airport staff/employees					
Employees		female	4		42-52
		male	2		26,40
	Employees Sum			6	26-52
Customs officer		female	1		26
		male	3		36-50
	Customs officer Sum			4	26-50
Special care services		female	2		27,59
		male	1		55
	Special care services Sum			3	27-59
Subtotal				13	26-59
	Total			101	14-79

Table 2: Direction of passengers after arriving to destination (inbound)

Means of transportation	Direction	No.	Sum
Train	National	13	17
	International	4	
Aircraft	National	8	17
	International	9	
Car	National	4	4
	International	0	
unknown		2	2
Sum			*40*
Frankfurt City		10	*10*

Table 3: Fear level and information needs of passengers and airport employees/staff

		Outbound passengers (n=38)	Inbound passengers (n=50)	Airport staff (n=13)
Fear level	None (0)	14 (37%)	34 (68%)	1 (8%)
	Moderate (1-2)	14 (37%)	10 (20%)	5 (38%)
	High (3-4)	10 (26%)	6 (12%)	7 (54%)
Receipt of leaflet	Yes	26 (68%)	19 (38%)	6 (46%)
	No	12 (32%)	31 (62%)	7 (54%)
information needs	Yes	42 (71%)	17 (29%)	11 (85%)
	No	8 (28%)	21 (72%)	2 (15%)

Figure 1: Information need: fear level and inbound/outbound flight

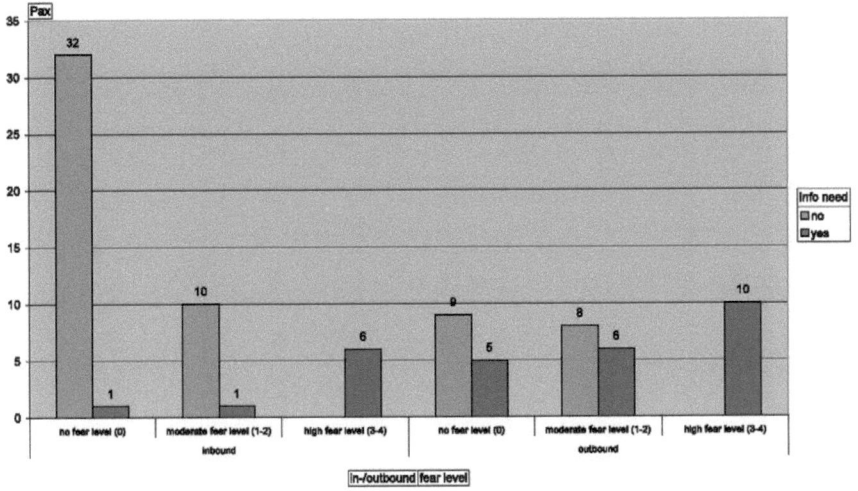

Acknowledgements

This book is a result of many people who have helped to make it real: first of all, I would like to thank Hubert Serve who has supported the idea from the beginning and who has given me the intellectual and institutional freedom to achieve my goal.

Simon Wessely has always been a supporting and inspiring adviser and I have learned a lot from his way to think about things. James Rubin is a genius – I adore his brilliant mind and it is an enriching pleasure to work with him.

Amy Iversen made my stay in London possible and I owe her a fortune for setting me into an intellectually stimulating and personally dedicated environment and looking after me so well.

Walter Gaber helped through the airport and security administration and gave important input to the airport study. Sabine Wicker is one of the most effective researchers I have ever known and I admire her for her strength and productivity – the airport study benefited a lot from her.

Hans-Reinhard Brodt gave me an institutional home and I am very grateful for his trust and support.

A very special thank goes to René Gottschalk. Without him – nothing would have been.

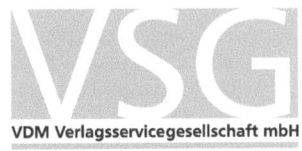

Die VDM Verlagsservicegesellschaft sucht für wissenschaftliche Verlage abgeschlossene und herausragende

Dissertationen, Habilitationen, Diplomarbeiten, Master Theses, Magisterarbeiten usw.

für die kostenlose Publikation als Fachbuch.

Sie verfügen über eine Arbeit, die hohen inhaltlichen und formalen Ansprüchen genügt, und haben Interesse an einer honorarvergüteten Publikation?

Dann senden Sie bitte erste Informationen über sich und Ihre Arbeit per Email an *info@vdm-vsg.de*.

Sie erhalten kurzfristig unser Feedback!

VDM Verlagsservicegesellschaft mbH
Dudweiler Landstr. 99
D - 66123 Saarbrücken

Telefon +49 681 3720 174
Fax +49 681 3720 1749

www.vdm-vsg.de

Die VDM Verlagsservicegesellschaft mbH vertritt

 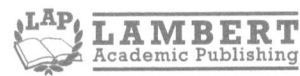 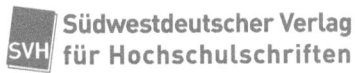

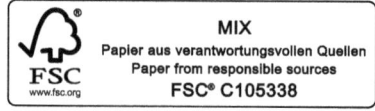

Printed by Books on Demand GmbH, Norderstedt / Germany